The Bach Flower Remedies

Illustrations and Preparations

Nora Weeks and Victor Bullen

The illustrations in the original book
were reproductions of water colours by
Marjorie Pemberton Piggott.
As these now illustrate *The Handbook of the Bach Flower Remedies*
rather than repeat them, we have chosen to include
photographs of the flowers.

SAFFRON WALDEN
THE C.W. DANIEL COMPANY LIMITED

First published in Great Britain by
The C.W. Daniel Company Limited
1 Church Path, Saffron Walden, Essex CB10 1JP, England
in 1964

© Nora Weeks and Victor Bullen 1964
Additional material and revisions © The Dr Edward Bach Centre 1990

ISBN 0 85207 205 8

Designed by Peter Dolton.

Design and Production in association
with Book Production Consultants, Cambridge, England.

Typeset by Anglia Photoset, Colchester.
Colour origination by Anglia Graphics, Bedford.
Printed and bound in Singapore by
Kyodo Printing Co (S'pore) Pte Ltd.

Contents

The Remedies

Acknowledgements

The photographs of Cerato, Chicory, Mustard, Olive, Pine, Red Chestnut, Rock Rose, Star of Bethlehem, Sweet Chestnut, Vine, Walnut, White Chestnut and Wild Rose were supplied by A–Z Botanical Collection Ltd., Hatfield, Herts., and we thank them for their assistance.

We would also like to thank Mechthild Scheffer for her photograph of Wild Oat on page 35.

All other photographs by Judy Howard of the Dr. Edward Bach Centre.

Preface

The last publication of this book was in the late seventies when it was withdrawn on the instruction of Nora Weeks in 1977 due to its misuse by certain groups overseas who took it as a licence to develop their own facsimiles of Dr. Bach's remedies. The following is an excerpt from a letter sent at that time to our publisher:

> *"We have decided not to send any more of the Illustrated Books to America, for many people are preparing them from the wrong flowers and preparing them in the wrong way, and selling them as Bach Remedies . . . and this we cannot have."*
>
> *Nora Weeks, 16th June 1977*

Now that Dr. Bach's work is so well known and respected throughout the world, it is our great pleasure to re-introduce this, the original book, describing the preparation of the Bach Flower Remedies as compiled by Dr. Bach's long-serving and devoted successors – Nora Weeks and Victor Bullen. It was their privilege to continue the Doctor's work of healing with the Flower Remedies and they did so for over forty years with true dedication. After Victor's death, Nora Weeks remained solely and entirely responsible for the future of Dr. Bach's work until her own passing in 1978. Her carefully appointed successors now carry on the hereditary duties accordingly, having also been empowered to determine, in their own time, the future curators of the Bach Centre and the doctor's work when it becomes their turn to stand down.

In offering this book we would emphasise that the descriptions and illustrations are sincerely provided for those who might enjoy the pleasure of preparing a remedy for themselves personally, although we cannot accept any responsibility for readers' own preparations. The following passages were written by Nora Weeks shortly before she died:

> *"We would like to emphasize that the book is essentially for those who wish to prepare their own essences from the actual wild flowers for their own use. We say 'for their own use' for if the essences or Stock bottles prepared from them are sold, it would be necessary to apply to the Department of Health and Social Security for a Manufacturer's Licence, this would entail much correspondence and a fee for the Licence. It would also take several years to prepare the 38 Remedies owing to the weather conditions and the time of flowering of the wild plants or trees.*
>
> *Most of our flowers have many varieties and care is necessary to select the right one. For instance there are many Willows – the Bach Willow, the golden osier, is difficult to distinguish, and the advice of a*

botanist is necessary. There are also various Centauries, Oaks, Mustard, Heather and Honeysuckles, amongst others. In the autumn of 1977 the Gentian amarella, the autumn Gentian was nowhere to be found in the usual places, due to the very dry summer of 1976 when the little plants died before their seeds had formed. We searched and searched until one day we thought at first glance we had found it. It was blue in colour with a white fringe at the base of the petals and much taller than usual as it was growing in quite long grass. However, it was the Gentian campestris, for our Gentian is purplish-blue with a dark fringe at the base of the petals. So you see, even after preparing Gentian amarella for over forty years we could have prepared it in error. There are eight different wild Gentians.

It is, as you see, vitally important to be sure you have the right flower and to prepare it in the right weather conditions. No cultivated or garden flowers must be used, but the wild flowers growing in the soil they choose themselves."

Nora Weeks

Some wild flowers, however, are scarce and so we implore anyone desirous of venturing into the making of a remedy to be most discerning and conscious of their responsibility to Nature. You will, we are sure, be aware of the Wildlife and Countryside Act which states that it is an offence to collect wild flowers without the landowner's permission, and even then certain species are protected unconditionally. Many wild flowers are sadly declining, especially those which rely annually on their seeds to flourish. Such flowers do not normally grow densely enough to propagate to any great extent and if the flower heads are taken under these conditions, the habitat of that plant becomes bereft of its continued presence. To pick wild flowers, therefore, just for the sake of experimentation would be unforgivable, so please be alert to the consequences of such action and choose those that grow in abundance such as the White Chestnut blossom instead of the delicate flowers of the meadow which are much less common. Those at the Bach Centre are acutely aware of their position and make every effort to conform to these important principles.

The Bach Flower Remedies have been made at the Bach Centre, Mount Vernon according to Dr. Bach's instructions, and with much loving care, since he made it his home and workplace in 1934, and many of his original locations are still used today in the preparation of the remedies.

Judy Howard and John Ramsell
Curators and Trustees of
The Dr. Edward Bach Healing Centre and Trust,
Mount Vernon, Sotwell.

Edward Bach

MB, BS, MRCS, LRCP, DPH

This book is dedicated to Edward Bach, physician, with the love and gratitude of those who knew and worked with him for many years, and in compliance with his wish that every detail of the knowledge he had gained for the alleviation of suffering and unhappiness should be freely available for everyone.

Edward Bach, born in Moseley, Warwickshire, in 1886, trained and qualified at University College Hospital, London, gaining the Diploma of Public Health at Cambridge in 1914. He then practised as consultant, bacteriologist and homoeopath for over sixteen years in London.

It was during his medical training that he first came to the conclusion that sickness and disease were not primarily due to physical causes, but to some deeper disharmony within the sufferer himself. That distress of mind, such as fear, worry, over-anxiety, impatience, so depletes the vitality of the individual that the body loses its natural resistance to disease and is then an easy prey to any infection, any form of illness.

These conclusions were strengthened and confirmed by Dr. Bach's observations during his sixteen years of medical practice, and in 1930 he determined to devote his whole time to the search for a simple method of treatment and harmless Remedies amongst the wild flowers of the countryside.

He gave up his big London practice and during the next seven years until his death in 1936, he perfected this system of healing and found thirty-eight Remedies, all, with one exception, the flowers of plants, trees and bushes.

With the help of the healing properties of these flowers, the sufferer can gain strength to overcome his anxieties, his fears and depressions, and so assist in his own healing, and can take the flower Remedies, if he wishes, at the same time as any other medicine or treatment.

Further information, advice and details of remedies and other books concerning Dr. Bach's work may be obtained from:

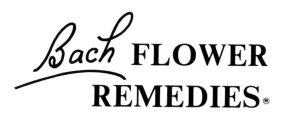

FLOWER REMEDIES®

The Dr. Edward Bach Centre,
Mount Vernon,
Sotwell, Wallingford,
Oxon. OX10 0PZ
England.

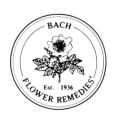

Introduction

The purpose of this book is to describe the two methods used in the preparation of the Bach Remedies.

The photograph facing the botanical description of each Remedy illustrates which part of the plant, tree or bush is used. The botanical descriptions are simple but, it is hoped, sufficient for the seeker to identify the plant. It should be remembered that colour and growth vary greatly with the soil, climate and conditions in which the plant is found, and also does the flowering time. The times are given for an average year.

With each remedy there is a brief indication of its use. The fuller description written by Dr. Edward Bach can be found in his booklet *The Twelve Healers and Other Remedies* which should always be referred to when selecting the Remedies.

It was Dr. Bach's great wish that all possible help should be given to those who would be using this system of medicine and we hope that this book will fulfil that wish.

Nora Weeks and Victor Bullen 1964

"We ask those living abroad not to prepare the Essences even if the flowers have the same Latin name for, due to the difference in soil and climate, they will not give the desired effect.

For those who live abroad where the English wild flowers do not grow, the book is only of interest in showing what the Bach flowers are like."

Nora Weeks

Solomon in all his glory was not arrayed like one of these.

Matthew 6.28

The Mother Tinctures

There are three stages in the preparation of the Bach Remedies: the first preparation or Mother Tincture; the second preparation or Stock bottle; the third preparation or Treatment bottle.

There are also two methods of preparing the Mother Tinctures. The sun method and the boiling method. The sun method is used for the flowers blooming during the late spring and in the summer when the sun is at the height of its power. The boiling method is used for the flowers and twigs of the trees, bushes and plants, most of which bloom early in the year before there is much sunshine.

Before preparing any Tincture, the plant or tree should be checked with the illustration and the botanical description as there are several varieties of the following: Centaury, Elm, Gentian, Heather, Honeysuckle, Mustard, Oak, Pine, Rock Rose, Scleranthus, Star of Bethlehem and Willow.

There are also cultivated varieties of many of the Remedy flowers: Clematis, Cherry Plum, Gentian, Honeysuckle, Mimulus, Rock Rose, Star of Bethlehem. The *wild* flowers growing in their natural habitat only should be used, with the exception of Ceratostigma willmottiana (Plumbago), the Olive and the Vine. The two latter should be prepared in warmer countries, such as the South of France, Italy or Spain.

The times of blooming will vary slightly according to the weather during that part of the year.

For the sun method of preparation, the flowers should be picked about 9 a.m., for the sun is gaining in power during the three hours between then and 12 noon. The flowers will already have been bathed in sunshine for some hours, and the blooms freshly opened and at their most perfect before the bees and flies and breezes have finished their work of spreading the pollen.

For the boiling method of preparation, a fine sunny morning should also be chosen and the flowers and twigs gathered about 9 a.m. for the same reason.

The flowers should be gathered from as many trees, plants and bushes of the same kind as possible.

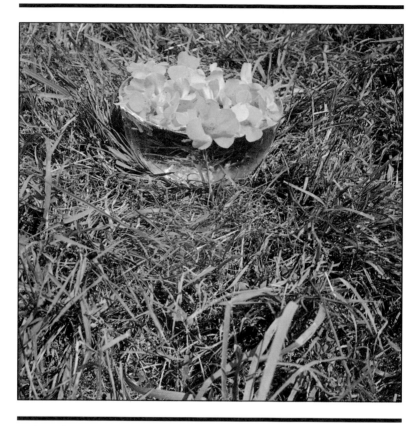

Sun Method – Mimulus

The Sun Method

Requirements

1. One thin, plain glass or crystal bowl, the size of a sugar bowl, to hold about half a pint of water. Not cut glass or oven glass.

2. One small jug, glass or china.

3. A one ounce dropper bottle.

The bowl, jug and bottle should first be sterilized, placed in cold water in a saucepan and gently boiled for twenty minutes, then dried carefully. Wrap the bowl and jug in a clean cloth. When cold, half fill the one ounce bottle with brandy, put on the cap and label with the name of the Remedy to be prepared and "Tincture".

4. One empty ½ pint sterilized bottle to be filled with bottled mineral or spring water should there be no clear unpolluted stream near the site where the flowers grow.

Method

Decide beforehand upon the field or hill-top where the plants, trees or bushes are growing, and choose a cloudless sunny morning. Take the bowl, jug, bottle and the one containing the water to this site before 9 a.m.

Place the bowl on the ground near the flowering plants, away from any tall grasses, bushes or trees which might cast a shadow over the bowl as the sun travels across the sky.

Fill the bowl to the brim with water from a nearby clear pure stream, or from the bottle you have brought with you.

Place a broad leaf, preferably from the plant you are preparing, on the palm of the hand and then pick the flower-heads just below the calyx, or the flowering spikes, from as many plants or bushes of the same kind as possible. Quickly float them on the surface of the water in the bowl and repeat this until the whole surface is thickly covered, overlapping the flowers, but seeing that each touches the water. Avoid casting a shadow over the bowl as you do this, or touching the water with your fingers.

Make a note of the time and leave the bowl in full sunshine for three hours.

At the end of this time and with a stalk from the plant you are preparing, remove the flower-heads, again avoiding touching the water with the fingers.

Pour the now vitalized water into the jug and fill the remaining half of the labelled bottle containing the brandy. Replace cap securely.

The Tincture will retain its strength indefinitely, and is the one from which Stock bottles are prepared (see page 96). If the Tincture is kept for several years, a slight sediment may form at the bottom of the bottle, this is not harmful. The liquid can be filtered into another sterilized bottle and relabelled.

List of Remedies Prepared by the Sun Method

These flowers are prepared by the sun method, with the best month in which to prepare them. The date will vary, however, from year to year according to the weather.

Oak

Indication: for the depression suffered by those
brave people who fight strongly against adverse conditions
without losing hope.

Quercus robur. The common oak.

Tree: deciduous, 60 to 80 feet high, with a massive trunk and grey-brown, thick, rough and deeply furrowed bark. The branches are many, tortuous and spreading. The twigs are greyish, bent and end in dense clusters of small blunt light brown and scaley buds.

Leaves: two to four inches long, short-stalked and oval in shape, dark green above and greyish-green beneath. They are alternate and deeply lobed, each lobe being rounded at the tip and with two folded ear-like lobes at the leaf-base.

Flowers: both male and female are borne on the same tree. The male catkins form loose drooping clusters, one to one and a half inches long, and are yellowish in colour, usually borne on the previous year's shoots. The female flowers are fewer and more inconspicuous, hidden amongst the leaves. They grow from the upper leaf axils of the new shoots, and occur in groups of two to five on a short erect stalk. They are formed of a cup-shaped calyx of a number of overlapping scales enclosing an ovary with three crimson styles. The calyx scales later form the cup for the acorn.

Blooms: with the young leaves in late April and May, according to the season. The Oak grows commonly in woods, hedgerows and meadows.

Prepare: by the sun method. Choose a field near a grove of Oaks and gather the *female* catkins only from as many different trees as possible, first covering the palm with a broad leaf to protect the flowers from the warmth of the hand. Cover the surface of the water in the bowl with the flowers.

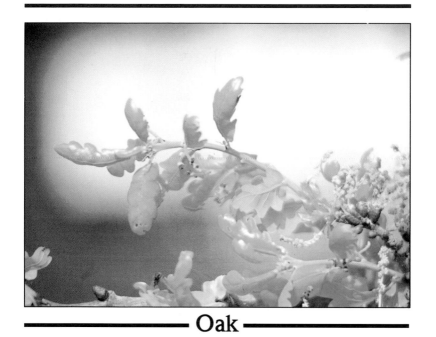

Oak

Oak – Quercus robur

Gorse

Indication: for very great hopelessness

Ulex europaeus. Whin, the common furze.

Shrub: an evergreen, two to eight feet high, spreading. The main branches are hairy and from them spring horizontally numerous short branches, grey-green in colour, furrowed and armed with many rigid, sharp and branched spines.

Leaves: are soft and hairy in the seedling, but as the bush matures, they become the sharply pointed linear green spines, half to three quarters of an inch long.

Flowers: are golden-yellow and abundant, formed like those of the pea family, and are produced singly from the leaf-axils of the previous year's shoots on hairy stalks, three quarters of an inch long. The corolla has five petals, the upper or standard petal is bilobed at the apex, the two wing petals are hairy on the lower surface, and the two keel petals are also hairy. The ten stamens are united to a sheath. The calyx is formed of two sepals, large and covered with blackish hairs outside, with two ovate bracts at the base. The flower is scented during the summer and autumn.

Blooms: most abundantly in April and May, although it begins to flower in February, with odd blooms at all times. It grows abundantly on stony soil, dry exposed commons and heaths.

Prepare: by the sun method in April, May or June. Choose big clumps of bushes and pick the flowers by the hairy stalk from the bushes in the centre and round the circumference of the clump so that the flowers from as many bushes as possible are gathered. Cover the palm of the hand with a broad leaf, and thickly cover the surface of the water in the bowl with the blooms.

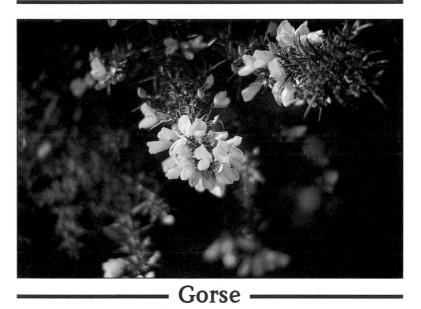

Gorse

Ulex europaeus

White Chestnut

*Indication: for persistent worrying thoughts
and mental arguments*

Aesculus hippocastanum. The Horse Chestnut.

Tree: 80 to 100 feet in height, with a grey brown scaly bark and stout arching branches which turn up at the tips in winter. On the smaller branches are the horseshoe markings which are the scars of last year's leaf-stalks. The twigs in winter are smooth and light brown with large sticky buds in opposite pairs. The terminal bud is larger than the lateral ones and contains both the leaf and the flower. Each bud is covered with fourteen overlapping scales protected by a resinous substance. The buds swell in early spring, the outer scales fall flat, the shoot within lengthens, the folded leaves at the top are covered with down which is thrown off as the leaves expand.

Leaves: as the leaflets emerge they droop and then expand, and when fully developed are large and fan-shaped. They are divided at the base into five or seven leaflets of different sizes with finely toothed margins.

Flowers: may be single or double and grow in dense erect spikes, the lower flowers having longer stalks thus forming a pyramid. The bell-shaped light green calyx has five lobes, the corolla five, six or seven petals, crinkled and pure white, splashed and dotted with crimson and yellow towards the base of the upper petal. The five to eight stamens are strongly curved, with a longer curved style. The upper flowers are usually male, the lower ones female.

Blooms: in late May and early June.

Prepare: by the sun method. Pick the male and female flowers (double or single) by their stalks from as many trees as possible, and cover the surface of the water in the bowl thickly with the blooms.

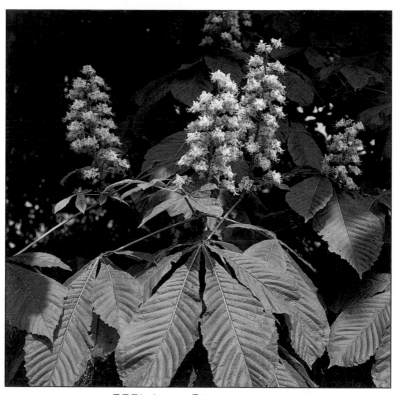

— White Chestnut —
Aesculus hippocastanum

Water Violet

Indication: for the quiet self-reliant people
who tend at times to be too proud
and aloof.

Hottonia palustris. Water Violet.

Plant: growing in water, and belonging to the Primrose family, not to the violets or pansies.

Leaves: are many in number forming a rosette at the base of the vertical flower stem. They are finely divided like a feather. This rosette serves to maintain the erect position of the flowering stem above the water, the leaves being submerged.

Flowers: are pale lilac with a yellow eye, and arranged in whorls one above the other round a leafless stalk. The flower-stalks have linear bracts, and curve downwards when the seeds are forming. The calyx has five narrow lobes, the petals are five-lobed, joined at the base. The five stamens are arranged opposite the lobes of the corolla and are attached to the tube.

Blooms: in early summer, May and June, growing in slow-moving streams, pools and ditches.

Prepare: by the sun method. Gather the flowers by their stalks from as many different plants as possible, and cover the surface of the water in the bowl with them. It is useful to have a walking-stick with a crook handle to draw the plants gently to the bank as they often grow well out in the stream.

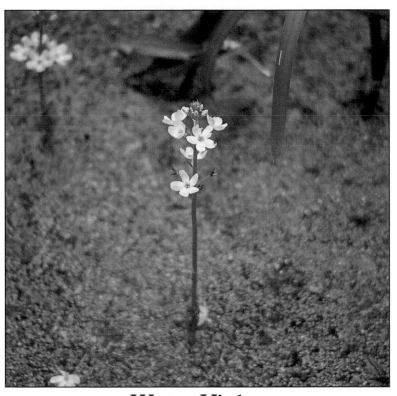

Water Violet

Hottonia palustris

Mimulus

*Indication: for the known fears of
everyday life – fear of people, of animals
of the dark, etc.*

Mimulus guttatus. The Monkey flower.

Plant: perennial, about a foot in height with a hollow stem.

Leaves: are rounded, opposite, toothed and smooth. At the base, the broad leaf stem is connected with that of the opposite leaf. There are several veins which run lengthwise.

Flowers: are yellow in colour, large and solitary, growing from the axils of the upper leaves on a flower stalk up to an inch and a half long. The corolla tube opens out into five large spreading lobes, the two upper ones slightly smaller than the three lower ones. The lower lip is more or less marked with small purple or reddish spots at the mouth of the tube. There are four stamens surrounding the pistil. The calyx is leafy and bell-shaped and five lobed.

Blooms: from June to August, in and near streams and brooks and in wet places. It is a naturalized plant in England and belongs to the same family as the Musk (Mimulus moschatus).

Prepare: by the sun method. Gather the flowers by their stalks from as many plants as possible, first covering the palm with a broad leaf to protect the delicate flowers from the warmth of the hand. Cover the surface of the water in the bowl with the blooms. Cultivated garden plants should never be used.

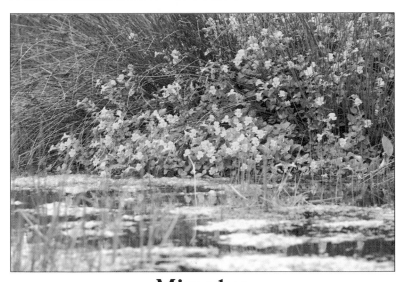

Mimulus

Mimulus Guttatus

Agrimony

*Indication: for those who hide their worries
from others under a cloak of cheerfulness and
good humour.*

Agrimonia eupatoria or **Agrimonia odorata.** Agrimony.

Plant: herbaceous, perennial, two to three feet high, and covered with soft hairs. Deep green in colour.

Leaves: are divided up to the mid-rib into coarsely toothed leaflets, oblong and ovate in shape, with alternate smaller leaflets between, and large leafy stipules at the base. Downy above and more densely so beneath.

Flowers: small and yellow on long tapering leafless spikes. Each flower is attached by a short stalk of its own and each blooms for three days. The lower buds open first. There are five petals and ten to fifteen stamens. The calyx is spiny with five overlapping scales. The flowers face upwards and outwards, but when they wither, the calyx points downwards and becomes woody and bell-shaped. The spines harden and the bristles hook on to the clothes of passers-by or to the coats of animals and by this means are distributed.

Blooms: from June to August, growing commonly in fields, hedge-banks and all waste places.

Prepare: by the sun method. Pick the flowering spike and end buds above any faded or dead flowers from as many plants as possible, first covering the palm with a broad leaf. Cover the surface of the water in the bowl with the blooms. Choose young plants where there are not too many unopened buds above the fully opened flowers.

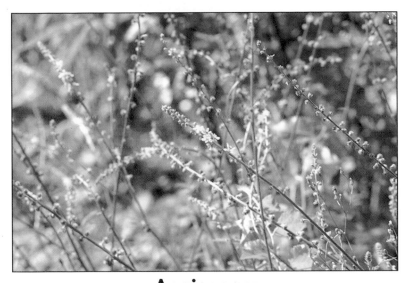

Agrimony
Agrimonia eupatoria

Rock Rose

Indication: for extreme fear, terror, panic

Helianthemum nummularium. Rock Rose.

Plant: perennial. A low spreading shrubby plant with short much branched woody stems which trail on the ground. Branchlets are produced annually up to a foot long.

Leaves: these are narrow, oblong and opposite, shortly stalked and entire. They are green above and white beneath and covered with branched hairs. The stipules are long and slender.

Flowers: bright yellow in colour, growing in terminal racemes, the lower flowers blooming first, and usually only one or two at a time. The blooms are quickly over when the flower-stalks bend downwards. The petals are five in number, soft and crumpled. The sepals are also five, three large and two small ones. The stamens surrounding the pistil are numerous.

Blooms: from June to September and grows on chalky downs, limestone and gravelly soils. It is said to be unknown in Ireland. The many coloured cultivated rockery plants are not used.

Prepare: by the sun method. First cover the palm with a broad leaf to protect the delicate flowers by the flower-stalks, a few at a time from as many plants as possible. Place quickly on the surface of the water.

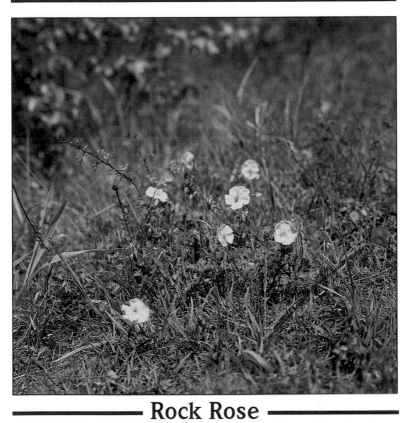

Rock Rose

Helianthemum nummularium

Centaury

*Indication: for those who lack the will-power
to refuse the demands of others and so
become willing slaves.*

Centaurium umbellatum. Centaury.

Plant: annual, varying between two and eighteen inches high according to habitat, with a square erect stem, much branched above and terminating in flat divided tufts of small rose-coloured flowers.

Leaves: are oblong, slender and opposite, smooth and pale green with three strong parallel ribs. The leaves have no stalks (sessile), and the root leaves often form a rosette.

Flowers: small and rose-pink, star-like. The corolla is funnel-shaped and five-cleft. The calyx of narrow sepals is also five-cleft. The stamens are five and the anthers become spirally twisted after the flower opens, which it only does in fine weather.

Blooms: from June to August in dry fields, waste places and road-sides.

Prepare: by the sun method. Pick the small tufts of flowers from as many plants as possible, first covering the palm with a broad leaf. Place quickly on the water in the bowl until the surface is completely covered.

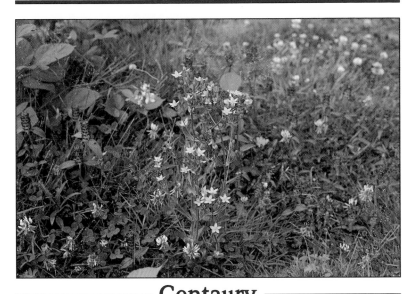

Centaury

Centaurium umbellatum

Scleranthus

*Indication: for those who cannot make up
their minds between two things. They do not
seek the advice of others.*

Scleranthus annuus. The annual Knawel.

Plant: small, bushy or procumbant, two to four inches high with numerous tangled stems.

Leaves: are awl-shaped, opposite and small, green, darker or lighter according to the soil in which the plant grows.

Flowers: are also pale or darker green in colour and grow either in the forks of the stems or in terminal tufts. There are no petals but a five cleft calyx, the pointed sepals being whitish at the edges, and contracted at the mouth of the tube. There are ten stamens and two styles.

Blooms: from July to September in wheat fields and sandy and gravelly soils.

Prepare: by the sun method. Pick the flowering stems and leaves from as many plants as possible, protecting the blooms from the warmth of the hand by a broad leaf. Cover the surface of the water in the bowl thickly with the flowering stems.

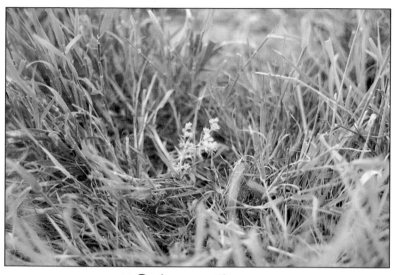

Scleranthus

Scleranthus annuus

Wild Oat

*Indication: dissatisfaction and uncertainty
in those who are talented but cannot
determine their course in life.*

Bromus ramosus. Hairy or Wood Brome-grass.

Grass with an erect hairy unbranched culm (stem) from two to six feet long.

Leaves: are green, broad and flat, long, drooping and finely pointed, the lower leaves are hairy. The tubular sheaths of the leaves clasp the main stem and are covered with long reflexed hairs.

The flower head (or panicle): at the top of the main stem is formed of many fine pendulous branches, usually in pairs, and from each of these branches arise two to four stemmed spikelets which are composed of overlapping scales. The two outer scales, called glumes, are bracts at the base of the spikelet, unequal in size and rounded at the back (keeled). The shorter glume is sharply pointed and has one nerve, the longer glume or bract is three to five nerved and bluntly pointed. The inner two scales, the lemma and the palea, enclose the bisexual flower. The lemma is oblong-lanceolate in shape, firm with a narrow membranous margin, with short hairs at the back. It is seven nerved and has a fine straight needle-like appendage (the awn) arising just below the apex. The lemma closely embraces the shorter scale, the keeled palea, and hidden at the base of these two scales is the flower, with two small scales enclosing the stamens, ovary and two feathery pistils.

Blooms: in July and August, and grows in damp woods, hedgerows, thickets and by roadsides. Widespread in the British Isles.

Prepare: by the sun method. Pick the flowering spikelets when in full pollen from many grasses, and cover the surface of the water in the bowl thickly.

The bromus ramosus does not look like the cultivated oat in appearance, and it may be difficult to identify.

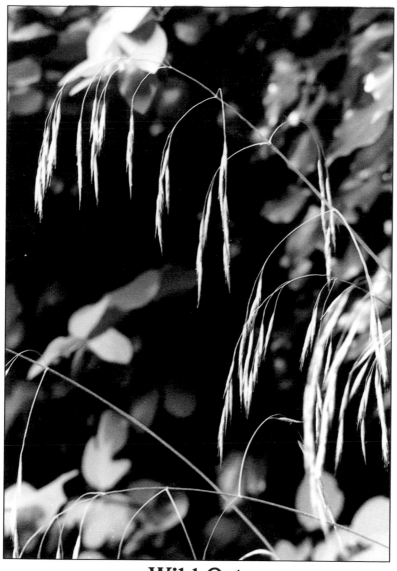

Wild Oat

Bromus ramosus

Impatiens

Indication: impatience and irritability.

Impatiens glandulifera. Policeman's Helmet.

Plant: annual, succulent and growing up to six feet or more in height. The stems are strong, green or crimson, ribbed and hollow, almost translucent. The side stems branch from swollen joints.

Leaves: are green and smooth with sharply toothed edges and a crimson mid-rib, with a pair of large stalked glands at the base of the leaf-stalk. The leaves are alternate, the ones beneath the flowers are crowded, stalked, broadly lanceolate and pointed, four to six inches long and two and a half inches broad.

Flowers: grow in stalked short whorls which cluster among the uppermost leaves. The bud bracts are ovate, pale crimson and soon fall off. The sepals are three in number and also pale crimson, two of them being obliquely ovate with a prominent mid-rib which is prolonged into a free tip. The third forms a large wide tube with a spine at the base. The corolla is formed of three petals, the upper one like the standard of the pea-flower, the other two irregular in shape, forming a lip in the front of the flower. All are mauve, some pale mauve and some crimson mauve. There are five stamens crowding round the ovary.

Blooms: from July to September and grows on river and canal banks and in low-lying damp soil.

Prepare: by the sun method. Use only the *pale mauve* flowers. Pick each flower separately by its stalk from many different plants, covering the palm with a broad leaf first, and cover the surface of the water in the bowl completely.

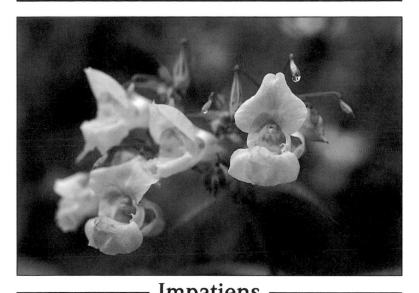

Impatiens

Impatiens glandulifera

Chicory

Indication: for those who are possessive and over-critical of others.

Chicorium intybus. Wild Succory.

Plant: a perennial with a tap-root, growing two to three feet high. The tough erect stem is grooved and hairy and has many lateral branches.

Leaves: the root-leaves spread out like a rosette on the ground, they are large and thickly covered with hairs, toothed like the dandelion leaves. The stem-leaves are very much smaller, the upper ones bract-like, the bases clasping the stem.

Flowers: are bisexual and generally grow in clusters of two or three in the axils of the stem-leaves and are stalkless. Usually only a few flowers bloom at the same time. They are composed of two or three rows of bright blue bracts, strap-shaped with a five notched straight end. The outer row of bracts is shorter than the inner one. The stamens and styles are also blue in colour.

Blooms: from July to September and grows on gravel, chalky and waste land, and the open borders of roadsides and fields.

Prepare: by the sun method. These flowers are very sensitive and fade quickly when picked, so cover the palm well with a broad leaf to protect them from the warmth of the hand. Pick two or three flowers only at a time and quickly float them on the surface of the water before gathering more from as many plants as possible.

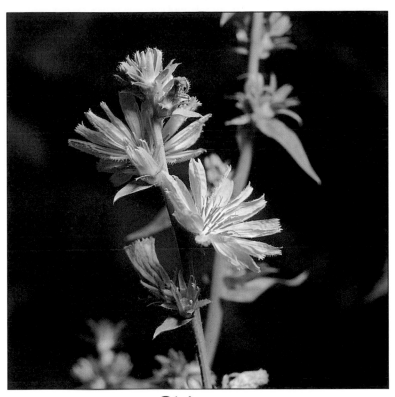

Chicory

Chichorium intybus

Vervain

*Indication: for the strain and tension felt
by those over-enthusiastic people who have fixed
and rigid ideas.*

Verbena officinalis. Vervain.

Plant: a perennial growing a foot or two high, with a tough erect and branching stem. The stem is four angled and sparsely covered with short hairs.

Leaves: are opposite and lanceolate, deeply cut and coarsely toothed, with short hairs on both surfaces.

Flowers: are small, pale mauve or lilac, they grow on slender terminal and auxillary spikes. The lower buds open first. The corolla tube divides into five unequal lobes, and white hairs at the mouth of the tube hide the four stamens. The calyx is also five lobed.

Blooms: from July to September and grows by the roadside, in dry waste places and sunny pastures.

Prepare: by the sun method. Gather the flowering spikes above any fading or dead flowers from as many plants as possible. Choose the younger plants so that there are not too many unopened buds above the fully opened flowers. Cover the surface of the water in the bowl completely.

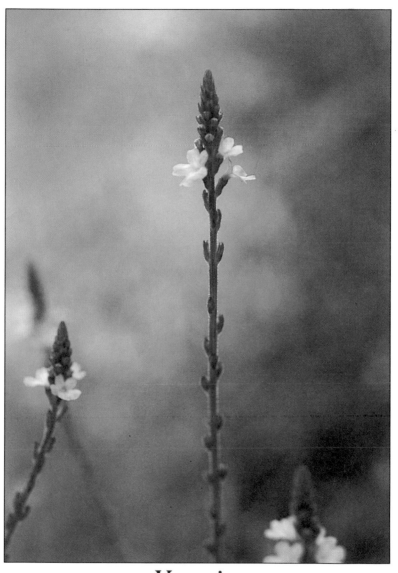

Vervain

Verbena officinalis

Clematis

Indication: for the day-dreamers who lack sufficient interest in the present.

Clematis vitalba. Travellers' Joy. Old Man's Beard.

Shrub: perennial, deciduous, a straggling woody climber over hedges and banks. The stems when old are thick and rope-like and covered with loose stringy pale brown bark.

Leaves: are opposite and compound, six to eight inches long with three to five oval irregular-toothed leaflets in pairs and a terminal one. The leaf-stalks are long and twisting, by means of which the shrub climbs.

Flowers: are in large panicles on the ends of the short auxillary branchlets. There are no petals but four to six thick downy sepals about half an inch long, tongue-shaped and petal-like, greenish-white in colour. These surround a cluster of creamy white stamens and pale green styles. The sepals curve downwards and outwards as the flower matures, and the styles elongate in autumn into long silvery thread-like tails, giving the plant the name of Old Man's Beard.

Blooms: in July, August and September, growing in hedges, thickets and woods on chalky soil and limestone.

Prepare: by the sun method. Gather the separate flowers by their stalks from as many different shrubs and parts of shrubs as possible, and cover the surface of the water in the bowl entirely.

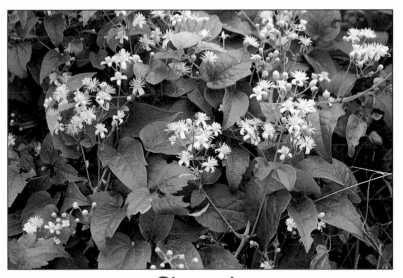

Clematis
Clematis vitalba

Heather

*Indication: for the talkative self-absorbed people
who fear loneliness.*

Calluna vulgaris. Ling. Scotch Heather.

Plant: shrubby and much branched, grows to about two feet high. The stems are rough and wiry and the branches are covered with very short soft hairs.

Leaves: these are small and opposite, and are arranged in four densely packed rows along the branches.

Flowers: mauve-pink in colour, occasionally white, are arranged in leafy spikes (racemes). The corolla is deeply four-lobed and concealed by the longer calyx. There are eight stamens and a long pistil which protrudes beyond the calyx. The calyx consists of four sepals, mauve-pink like the corolla, dry and rough. Below it there are four small triangular bracts fringed with soft hairs and a short flower stem.

Blooms: from July to September on heaths, dry moors, and open barren places. It should not be confused with the pinky-red Bell Heather (Erica cinerea).

Prepare: by the sun method. Gather the freshly flowering sprays and leaves, above any dead or faded flowers from plants round the circumference and the centre of the heather patch, and place quickly on the surface of the water in the bowl.

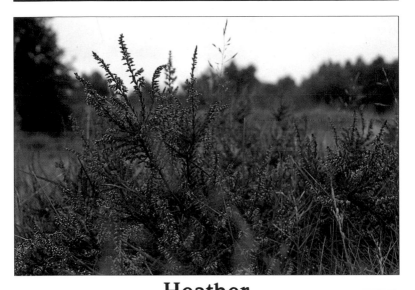

Heather

Calluna vulgaris

Cerato

*Indication: for those who do not trust
their own decisions and repeatedly seek
the advice of others.*

Ceratostigma willmottiana. Plumbago.

Shrub: deciduous, two to four feet high, a native of Tibet, China, the Himalayas. The young stems are angled and sometimes reddish.

Leaves: alternate, stalkless, lanceolate, from one to two inches long and bristly on both surfaces.

Flowers: are packed closely in terminal heads, opening successively from the axils of slender lanceolate pointed bracts, edged with stiff bristles. The corolla is slender, a pale blue tube, three quarters of an inch long, with five spreading petals, bright blue in colour, white at the base. The stamens are slender filaments attached to the tube opposite each petal. The anthers are purple in colour. The calyx is five-lobed and awl-shaped.

Blooms: August and September in gardens. This is a cultivated plant in England, there is no wild variety.

Prepare: by the sun method. Choose your flowers from a country garden and pick the single blooms just below the calyx from two or more shrubs if possible, first covering the palm with a broad leaf to protect the delicate flower from the warmth of the hand. Place quickly on the surface of the water in the bowl until it is completely covered.

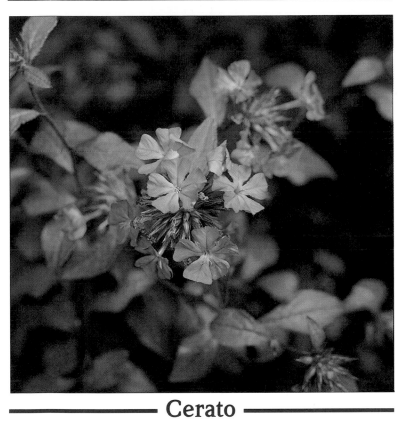

Cerato

Ceratostigma willmottiana

Gentian

Indication: for doubt and discouragement.

Gentiana amarella. Felwort. The autumn Gentian.

Plant: with square, leafy and erect stems, branched or simple, and tinged with crimson or purple, six inches to a foot high.

Leaves: are dark green with three prominent veins, opposite and generally stalkless (sessile). They clasp the stem at the base and are lanceolate in shape.

Flowers: are numerous, single or in clusters and purplish-blue in colour, growing on short stalks in the axils of the leaves. There is one terminal flower at the top of the stem. The corolla-tube is twice as long as the calyx and divides into five lobes with a dense fringe of erect, stiff purple hairs at the mouth of the tube. The calyx is also five-cleft, narrow and acutely pointed and of equal size. The stamens are five and alternate with the five corolla lobes. There is one style and two stigmas.

Blooms: from August to October, on dry hilly pastures, cliffs and dunes.

Prepare: by the sun method. Gather the flowers just below the calyx from as many plants as possible, first covering the palm with a broad leaf. Place quickly on the water in the bowl until the surface is completely covered.

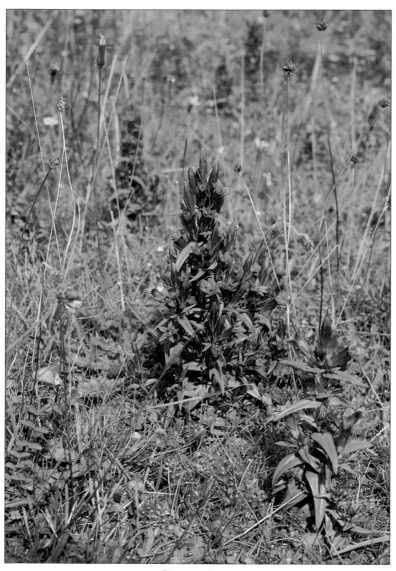

Gentian

Gentiana amarella

Olive

Indication: for complete mental exhaustion.

Olea europaea. Olive.

Tree: a small evergreen, 30 to 40 feet high, with many thin branches. The bark is pale grey in colour.

Leaves: are opposite and lanceolate, leathery and about two and a half inches long. They are entire, acute and smooth, silvery beneath and pale green above.

Flowers: are borne in clusters or racemes, small and inconspicuous, 20 to 30 flowers to each inflorescence, arising from the axils of the leaves. The corolla tube is short and divides into four petals, whitish in colour and spreading. The two stamens are attached to the corolla tube. The ovary is divided into two cells, the style is short and the stigma bilobed. The calyx is cup-shaped and very shortly four-toothed.

Blooms: in spring, according to the climate of the country where the tree grows.

Prepare: by the sun method. Cover the palm with a broad leaf to protect the delicate flowers from the heat of the hand, and pick the flower clusters from as many trees as possible. Place them quickly on the water, covering the whole surface.

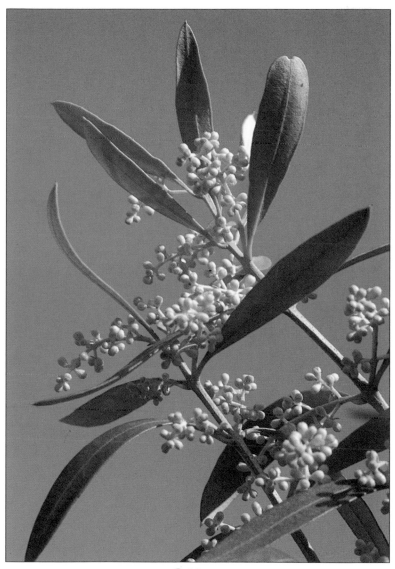

Olive

Olea europaea

(Before the flowers have burst forth)

Vine

*Indication: for those efficient strong-minded
people who are inclined to be dominent
and force their will upon others.*

Vitis vinifera. Grape vine.

Shrub: a deciduous and long-lived tendril climbing shrub, 50 feet or more in length with woody stems.

Leaves: these are three to five inches wide, three to five lobed and coarsely toothed, growing alternately, with small stipules at the base. The tendrils, which help in supporting the shoots, arise opposite two-thirds of the leaves.

Flowers: grow in dense clusters and are small, green and fragrant. There are five petals which unite at the tips forming a cap which is pushed off when the stamens are ripe. The calyx is small, forming a rim at the base of the petals and is five-lobed or toothed. The five stamens are opposite the petals. The berry is the grape.

Blooms and grows in warmer countries and the time of flowering varies with the climate.

Prepare: by the sun method. Pick the flowering clusters when at their most perfect from as many different shoots of the vine as possible. Cover the surface of the water in the bowl with the blooms.

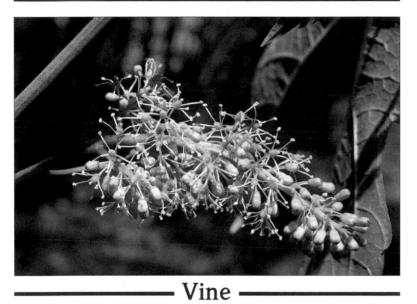

Vine

Vitis vinifera

Rock Water

*Indication: for those who practise too rigid
a self-discipline and are hard masters
to themselves.*

Rock Water.

This is the water taken from some well or spring known for its power to heal the sick.

Not the water of spas, well-known for their valuable medicinal properties, nor the wells and springs over which chapels and shrines have been built by man, but the half-forgotten spring or well, many of which are still to be found in various parts of the country, in its natural state, open to the sunshine and the air, amongst the trees or in the fields, or some village churchyard.

Prepare: by the sun method. Fill the glass bowl to the brim from the well or spring, place it on the ground in the sunshine for three hours on any perfect sunny day during the summer. The sun is at its greatest strength during the months of June and July.

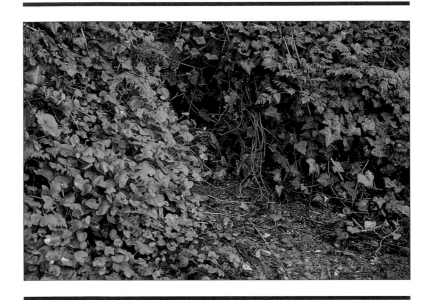

The Spring in Sotwell, a short walk from Mount Vernon.
It was first used to prepare the Rock Water remedy
by Dr. Bach who also found it contained healing properties
beneficial to the eyes.

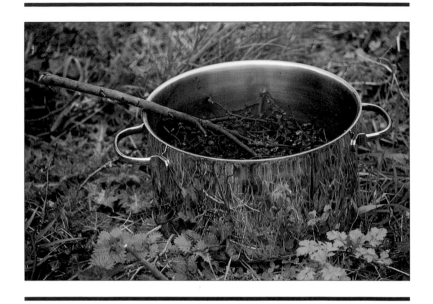

Preparation of Elm by boiling

The Boiling Method

Requirements

1. A six pint enamel or stainless steel saucepan and lid.

2. Two small china or glass jugs.

3. A one ounce dropper bottle.

These should first be sterilized. Place the jugs and bottle in the saucepan filled with bottled mineral or spring water and boil gently for twenty minutes. Then dry carefully and wrap the jugs in a clean cloth. When cold, half fill the bottle with brandy, put in the cork and label with the name of the Remedy to be prepared and "Tincture".

4. Two or three pieces of filter paper, obtainable from most chemists and supermarkets.

Method

Decide beforehand upon the wood, hedgerow or field where the trees, bushes or plants are growing. Choose a fine sunny morning, and before 9 a.m. take the saucepan, covered with its lid to keep out the dust, to the chosen spot.

Fill the saucepan three quarters full with the flowering sprays, leaves and twigs (about four ounces). Replace the lid and return home as quickly as possible. Cover the flowers and twigs with two pints of bottled mineral or spring water. Place the saucepan *without* its lid over the heat and bring the water to the boil, pressing the flowers beneath the water with a twig of the same bush or tree from time to time. Make a note of the time and boil for half an hour.

At the end of half an hour, remove the saucepan from the heat and stand out of doors until cold. When cold, remove all twigs, leaves and flowers with another twig of the same tree or bush to prevent the fingers from touching the water. Allow the saucepan to stand for a further period for the sediment to settle as much as possible.

Cover one of the jugs with filter paper. Fill the other jug carefully from the saucepan without disturbing the sediment, then pour the liquid a little at a time on to the filter paper. This process takes a long time. When sufficient quantity has been filtered, fill the remaining half of the bottle containing the brandy and replace cap securely.

With tree flowers and twigs there is often much sediment and it may be advisable to filter the liquid twice. Even then, after a time – some months – sediment may form at the bottom of the bottle, it should be refiltered and rebottled.

The Tincture will retain its strength indefinitely and is the one from which Stock bottles are prepared (see page 96).

List of Flowers Prepared by the Boiling Method

These flowers are prepared by the boiling method, with the best month in which to prepare them. The date will vary, however, from year to year according to the weather.

Cherry Plum

Indication: fear of the mind giving way.

Prunus cerasifera. Cherry Plum.

Tree or bush: 10 to 12 feet high, the young twigs usually thornless, commonly used as hedging and shelter-belts round orchards.

Leaves: are narrow, oval or obovate, half to two inches long and half to one inch wide. The edges are toothed and downy along the mid-rib and the veins beneath.

Flowers: are pure white, three quarters to one inch across, slightly larger than those of the sloe or blackthorn. They are usually produced singly, but sometimes grow two or three together on either side of the leaf-bud, and often form dense clusters on short spur-like twigs. The petals are five in number, the sepals also five, the stamens numerous. The flower stalks are quarter of an inch long. The fruit, which is not produced each year, is small, red and yellow and cherrylike.

Blooms: in early spring, February to April, before the leaves appear.

Prepare: by the boiling method. Pick the flowering twigs with the flowers about six inches long, from as many bushes as possible and place in the saucepan until it is three parts full.

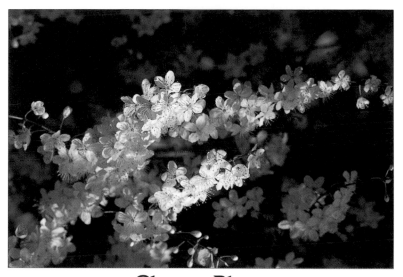

Cherry Plum

Prunus cerasifera

Elm

Indication: for those who, although fulfilling their work in life, become despondent at times feeling the responsibility is too great.

Ulmus procera. The English or common elm.

Tree: 60 to 150 feet high, with a massive trunk, deeply fissured greyish bark, and numerous spreading branches.

Leaves: are two to three and a half inches long, one and a half to two and a half inches broad, growing alternately, broadly oval with sharply toothed margins. The leaves are rough above and downy beneath with a short stalk.

Flowers: these bloom on the bare twigs before the leaves open. They are small and very numerous, in purplish-brown clusters. Each flower has a four-toothed bell-shaped calyx, no petals, four stamens and a one-celled ovary bearing two spreading hairy styles.

Blooms: from February to April according to the weather, in woods and hedgerows.

Prepare: by the boiling method. Pick the twigs with the flower-clusters about six inches in length, from as many trees as possible, sufficient to fill the saucepan three quarters full.

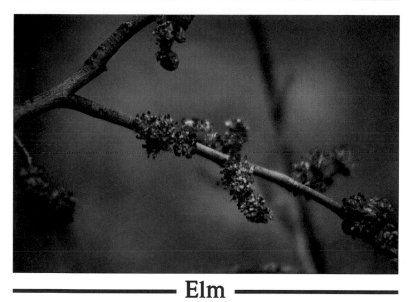

Elm

Ulmus procera

Aspen

Indication: for vague fears of unknown origin.

Populus tremula. Aspen.

Tree: rather slender, seldom more than 80 feet in height, with a smooth greyish bark, grey-brown twigs and slightly sticky glossy brown buds.

Leaves: are dark green, two to three inches wide, nearly circular in shape with a blunt pointed tip and bluntly toothed wavy edges. The leaves are woolly when young, but smooth in the autumn. The leaf-stalks are long and slender and flattened which causes the leaves to flutter and tremble in the slightest breeze.

Flowers: male and female catkins appear before the leaves on the same tree. The male catkin is two to three inches long, pendulous with brown hairy scales and reddish anthers. The female catkin is smaller, with a four-lobed purple stigma at the top of a roundish smooth ovary.

Blooms: in March and April, before the leaf-buds burst.

Prepare: by the boiling method. Gather both male and female catkins with about six inches of the twig and young leaf-buds from several trees, sufficient to fill the saucepan three quarters full.

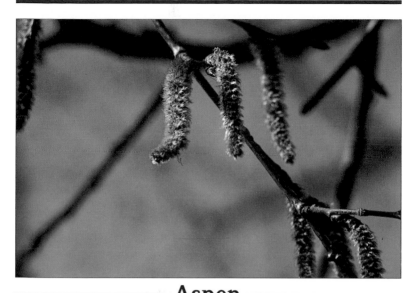

Aspen

Populus tremula

Beech

Indication: intolerance.

Fagus sylvatica. Beech.

Tree: 60 to 100 feet high, with a smooth silver-grey bark.

Leaves: the winter buds are long, slender and pointed with many closely overlapping brown scales which burst early in May at the same time as the flowers. The leaves are alternate, oval, smooth-faced with straight lateral veins, a pointed apex and slightly toothed margins. At first they are folded and covered with a soft silky down, later they become opaque and glossy.

Flowers: the male and female growing on the same tree and appearing with the leaves. The male flowers have no petals but four to six sepals covered with silky hairs surround eight to sixteen stamens. They cluster to form a hanging purplish-brown tassel on a long stalk. The female flower-clusters consist of two flowers with many stamens, and are enclosed in a cup of overlapping scales which later become the bristly "mast" protecting the beech-nut.

Blooms: April and May in woods.

Prepare: by the boiling method. Gather the young shoots with the newly opened leaves and the male and female flowers about six inches long from as many trees as possible, filling the saucepan three quarters full.

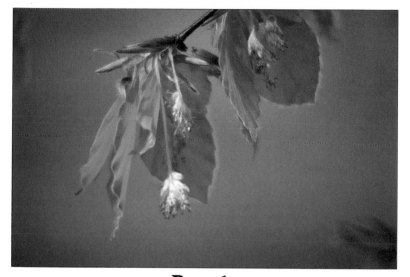

Beech
Fagus sylvatica

Chestnut Bud

*Indication: for those who are slow to learn
even from repeated experiences.*

Aesculus hippocastanum. The white chestnut. Horse chestnut.

Tree: 80 to 100 feet high, with a grey-brown scaley bark and stout arching branches which turn up at the tips. On the smaller branches are the horse-shoe markings which are the scars of last year's leaf-stalks. The twigs in winter are smooth and light brown with large sticky buds in opposite pairs. The terminal bud is larger than the lateral ones and contains both the leaf and the flower. Each bud is covered with fourteen overlapping scales protected by a resinous substance. The buds gradually swell in early spring, the outer scales fall flat, the shoot within lengthens, the folded leaves at the top are covered with down which is thrown off as the leaves expand.

It is at this stage that the Chestnut Bud is ready for preparing the Remedy. The time, April or May according to the weather. Make certain the trees are the white chestnut and not the red chestnut.

Prepare: by the boiling method. Pick the bud and about six inches of the twig from as many trees as possible, filling the saucepan three quarters full.

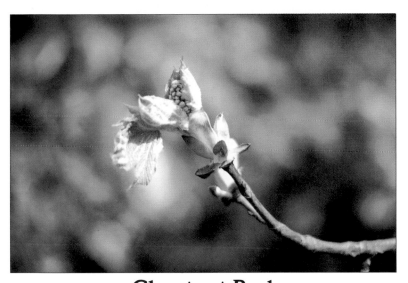

Chestnut Bud

Aesculus hippocastanum

Hornbeam

*Indication: for those who think they will not
have the strength to fulfil their
daily tasks.*

Carpinus betulus. Hornbeam.

Tree: 50 to 70 feet high, superficially resembling the beech tree. Its bark is smooth and light grey, its bole deeply fluted. When young, the tree is pyramidal in shape, but later is rounded with the branch-tips pendulous.

Leaves: in spring the new leaves are dark green, oval with doubly serrated edges, downy beneath and on the mid-rib above, one to three and a half inches long. They have a rounded or heart-shaped base and pointed apex. Each has ten to thirteen pairs of veins which run straight and parallel. They are short-stalked and alternate.

Flowers: male and female grow on the same tree, greeny-brown in colour. The male flowers grow in the axils of last year's leaves, and are long drooping cylindrical catkins with rounded scales, sharp-tipped, one and a half inches long. Three to twelve stamens are contained in each bract. The female flowers, growing at the end of short lateral shoots, are erect until the fruit forms, then they hang down. They are produced in pairs facing each other, and have three-lobed greenish scales, large and leaf-like which soon fall off. The middle lobe is one to one and a half inches long and is often toothed. There are two red stigmas.

Blooms: April and May in woods and coppices.

Prepare: by the boiling method. Pick the young twigs with the leaves, male and female flowers, about six inches long from as many trees as possible. Fill the saucepan three parts full.

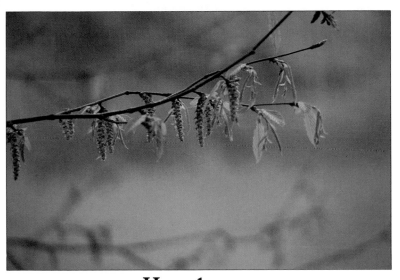

Hornbeam

Carpinus betulus

Larch

*Indication: for those who lack confidence
in themselves and fear failure.*

Larix decidua. Larch.

Tree: lofty with a straight tapering trunk, 80 to 100 feet high. The bark is brown and as the tree grows, it splits into deep longitudinal fissures. The lower branches are long and spreading with up-turned tips and pendulous greyish-yellow shoots.

Leaves: the drooping twigs bear bunches of 30 to 40 slender needle-like leaves in spreading tufts like brushes. These are bright green in spring, becoming deeper green as the year advances. The Larch is the only coniferous tree to lose its leaves in winter.

Flowers: both sexes grow on the same tree and appear when the leaves are just showing as small bright green tufts. The male flowers are cylindrical catkins about half an inch long, with a mass of golden yellow stamens cupped in a number of scales. The female catkins are conspicuous, bright red catkins, erect and almost cylindrical.

Blooms: in April and May according to the weather, and grows on hills and the outer edges of woods.

Prepare: by the boiling method. Pick about six inches of the twig with the young green leaf-tufts and the male and female flowers, and gather from as many trees as possible. Fill the saucepan three quarters full.

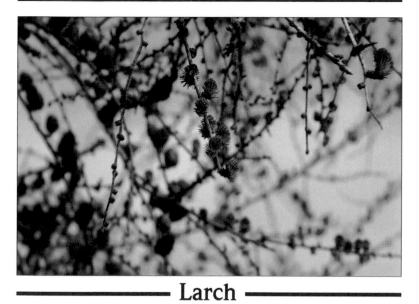

Larch

Larix decidua

Walnut

*Indication: for the definite people who at times
are led away from their own aims
and work by the strong opinions of others.*

Juglans regia. Walnut.

Tree: 40 to 100 feet high, with a big bole and huge spreading head. The bark is grey, smooth when young, but with deep longitudinal furrows forming as the tree matures, making it very rugged. The twisted branches take an upward turn.

Leaves: these appear late and are large with a variable number of smooth lance-shaped leaflets with slightly wavy edges in opposite pairs. The young shoots and leaves are reddish in colour.

Flowers: both male and female grow on the same tree. The male flower is a drooping catkin with a calyx of four to five scales, greenish in colour, enclosing a large number of stamens. The female flowers are solitary or a few grouped at the end of the shoot. They are few in number. The calyx, bottle-shaped, closely surrounds the ovary which has two or three fleshy stigmas. The flowers bloom before or just as the leaf-buds burst. The fruit is the edible walnut.

Blooms: in early spring, April and May, in hedgerows and orchards.

Prepare: by the boiling method, picking about six inches of the young shoot, leaves and *female* flowers from as many trees as possible. Fill the saucepan three parts full.

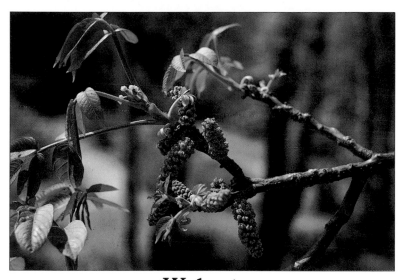

Walnut

Juglans regia

Star of Bethlehem

Indication: for shock.

Ornithogalum umbellatum. Star of Bethlehem.

Plant: closely allied to the onion and garlic, growing from a small bulb.

Leaves: these arise from the bulb and are long, very slender (like the leaves of the crocus), dark green with a white line down the centre.

Flowers: a leafless stalk grows from the centre of the bulb, six inches to a foot high, ending in the cluster or umbel of flowers. The central stalks of the umbel are longer than the outer ones. The flowers have no calyx but a star-like corolla of six petals, which are very white inside, with a green stripe down the outer surface. There are six stamens. The flowers open only in the sunshine.

Blooms: from April to May and grows in meadows and small woods.

Prepare: by the boiling method. Pick the flowering clusters when they are fully open, with a small piece of the main stem from as many plants as possible, filling the saucepan three parts full.

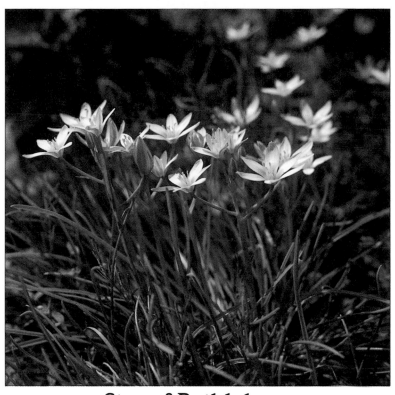

Star of Bethlehem

Ornithogalum umbellatum

Holly

Indication: for those who suffer from feelings
of envy, jealousy, revenge and suspicion.

Ilex aquifolium. Holly.

Tree or bush: a much branched evergreen with a silver-grey smooth trunk and deep green twigs.

Leaves: are short-stalked, alternate, oval and deeply lobed, each lobe ending in a sharp spine. They are two or three inches long, leathery, glossy and dark green above, dull and lighter green on the under surface. The upper leaves of the tree are often without spines.

Flowers: the male and female flowers usually grow on different bushes, but sometimes a bush may be found to be bisexual. The female flowers are small and white with short stalks, growing in the axils of the leaves. The petals are four in number, united into a short tube at the base. The four stamens are arranged alternately with the petals. The male flowers are similar, but have two to four stigmas forming a disc-like plate on the ovary. The fruit is the red berry.

Blooms: in May and June, in woods and hedgerows.

Prepare: by the boiling method. Pick the flowering twigs, female and/or male flowers, with a few of the leaves, about six inches long from as many bushes as possible. Fill the saucepan three parts full.

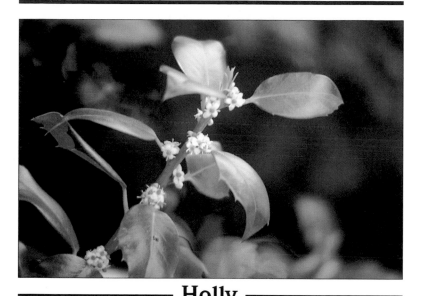

Holly

Ilex aquifolium

Crab Apple

*Indication: for those who have a feeling
of uncleanliness.*

Malus pumila. Crab Apple.

Tree or large bush: deciduous, low and spreading, 20 to 30 feet high, with a grey and crooked trunk, fissured and cracked. The branches are brown in colour and slightly drooping, with long shoots bearing the leaves and flowers in small clusters on dwarf rigid spurs.

Leaves: are alternate, oval with coarsely toothed margins, darker green and smooth above, paler and downy beneath, and about one and a half inches long.

Flowers: these grow in clusters of five or six with the leaves at the top of a short shoot. The buds are deep rose-pink, the petals, when open, are white tinted with pink, and are heart-shaped and five in number. The calyx is formed of five pointed lobes which are woolly within. Stamens number about 20.

Blooms: in May, according to the season, and grows in hedges, thickets and open woodlands.

Prepare: by the boiling method. Pick the rigid spurs with the leaves and flower clusters from as many trees as possible, filling the saucepan three parts full.

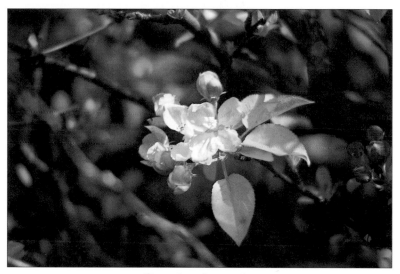

Crab Apple

Malus pumila

Willow

Indication: for resentfulness and bitterness.

Salix vitellina. The Yellow Willow. The Golden Osier.

Tree: often pollarded, whose bole is covered with a strong thick grey-brown bark, rough and deeply fissured. The twigs are flexible, smooth and resilient, and turn a bright orange-yellow in winter.

Leaves: grow alternately, are short stalked, narrow and lance-like, tapering to a slender tail-like point, two to four inches long. They are glossy green above and silky beneath, with edges faintly toothed.

Flowers: the catkins, male and female, grow on different trees, and are long and slender. They appear with the unfolding leaves and are pollinated chiefly by the wind.

Blooms: early in May and grows on moist and low-lying ground.

Prepare: by the boiling method. Pick the catkins, either sex, with about six inches of the twig and young leaves from as many trees as possible.

There are many varieties of the Willow tree, but the Salix vitellina (vitellina – like the yoke of an egg) can always be recognized by its brilliant yellow twigs in winter.

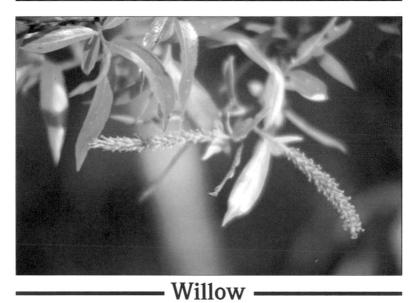

Willow

Salix vitellina

Red Chestnut

Indication: for fear and over-anxiety
for others.

Aesculus carnea. Red Chestnut.

Tree: smaller and less robust than the White or Horse Chestnut. The trunk is deeply furrowed with a greenish smooth bark which later becomes scaly. The buds are borne in opposite pairs in the axils of last year's leaves. The terminal ones are larger than the lateral buds, and are covered by large overlapping bud-scales, protected by a glutinous substance.

Leaves: as the leaves emerge they are covered with white down, the leaflet drooping until the leaf is fully expanded in early May. They are large, compound and formed by five or seven leaflets, broadening towards the tip then suddenly tapering to a point. The margins are serrated.

Flowers: these are in large upright inflorescences, pyramidal in shape as the lowest flowers have longer stalks. The corolla is formed of four or five petals of unequal size, the colour is pinky-red. There are five to eight stamens which have long curved filaments, and the style is also long and curved. The calyx is formed of five joined sepals.

Blooms: in late May and early June according to the season.

Prepare: by the boiling method. Gather about six inches of the twig with the flowering pyramid and young leaves, from as many trees as possible and fill the saucepan three quarters full.

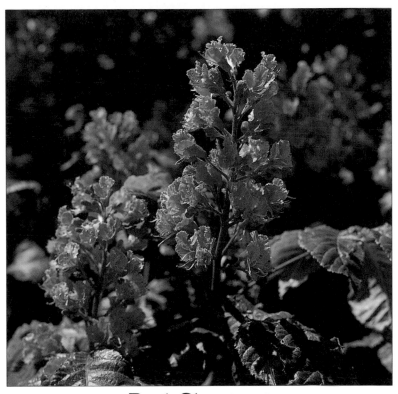

Red Chestnut

Aesculus carnea

Pine

Indication: for self-reproach.

Pinus sylvestris. Scots Pine.

Tree: an evergreen, growing up to a height of 100 feet, with a straight cylindrical trunk, a rough bark, the lower part being reddish-brown, the upper part and the branches orange-brown in colour. The branches are short and spreading.

Leaves: grow in pairs in dense tufts. They are from two to three inches long, slender and needle-like, grooved above and convex beneath. They appear at the ends of the pale brown scaley twigs and are surrounded at the base by a band of small scales. In the centre of each tuft is a cluster of golden brown resinous pointed buds. The leaves fall off every two or three years and are of a whitish-blue colour the first year, but become deep dark green later on.

Flowers: the male and female grow on the same tree. The golden-yellow male flowers are small and form clusters, abundantly covered with yellow pollen, at the top of the shorter shoots. The female flowers or cones, grow singly or in small clusters of three, red and egg-shaped, at the apex of the year-old shoots.

Blooms: in May and early June in pine woods and on heathland.

Prepare: by the boiling method. Pick about six inches of the young shoots together with the male and female flowers, and when the male flowers are in full pollen, from as many trees as possible. Fill the saucepan three parts full.

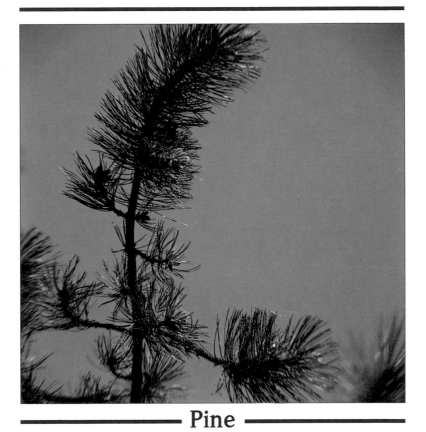

Pine

Pinus sylvestris

Mustard

*Indication: for the deep depression
and gloom for which no explanation
can be given.*

Sinapis arvensis. Charlock. Wild Mustard.

Plant: an annual, one to two feet high, with upright branched stems which are grooved and often covered with short rough hairs.

Leaves: the lower ones have short stalks, the upper ones are stalkless, rough and lyre-shaped with coarsely toothed edges and a few stiff hairs mostly on the lateral forked nerves. On the leaf-stalk below the larger leaves there are a few smaller leaves.

Flowers: are arranged at first in close racemes or clusters which soon elongate as the fruits are formed. The flower-stalks are very short. The corolla is formed of four petals, spoon-shaped with slender claws, which are bright yellow in colour. There are six stamens, four long and two short, with rather large anthers, arrow-shaped at the base. The spreading sepals of the calyx are four in number and soon fall off.

Blooms: in May, June and July in fields and way-sides.

Prepare: by the boiling method. Pick the flower-heads above the faded blooms and seed-pods from as many plants as possible, filling the saucepan three quarters full.

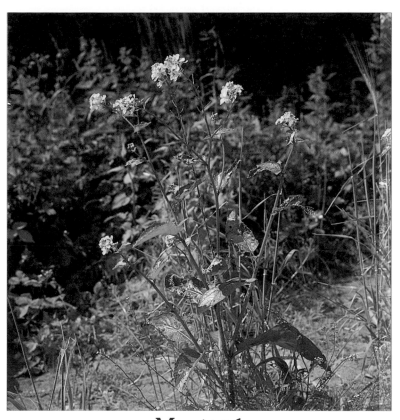

Mustard

Sinapis arvensis

Honeysuckle

Indication: for those whose thoughts dwell
too much upon memories, events and
happiness of the past.

Lonicera caprifolium. Honeysuckle.

Shrub or woody climber with a tough stem.

Leaves: are opposite and entire with no stipules. The lower leaves are stalked, the uppermost pairs are united by their bases round the stem, and are oblong in shape.

Flowers: grow in terminal heads or clusters. The corolla tube is one to two inches long and divides into five lobes which split into two opposite lips. The upper lip of four united lobes, the lower one a single lobe. There are five long and protruding stamens and a pale green pin-headed pistil. The outer surface of the petals is red or deep pink, the inner surface white, but on pollination the flower turns yellow. The calyx is small, the sepals are united, five-toothed and glandular.

Blooms: in June, July and August, in woods, hedgerows and heaths. The Lonicera caprifolium is more rare than the yellow-flowered Lonicera periclymenum, the common honeysuckle.

Prepare: by the boiling method. Pick the flowering clusters with about six inches of the stalk and leaves, from various parts of the shrub.

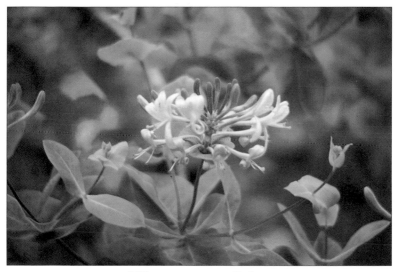

Honeysuckle

Lonicera caprifolium

Sweet Chestnut

Indication: extreme anguish in those who have reached the limit of their endurance.

Castanea sativa. The Spanish Chestnut. The edible chestnut.

Tree: deciduous, 60 to 80 feet high, with a grey-brown thick bark which is deeply furrowed longitudinally, and which, as the tree matures, begins to twist spirally around the trunk.

Leaves: are large, glossy, alternate, dark green above, rather downy beneath and about five to nine inches long, two and a half inches broad, with a short stalk. They are elliptical in shape, tapering to a point at each end. The margins are toothed with sharp spreading teeth.

Flowers: appear after the leaves, the male and female flowers growing on the same tree. The catkins are long, five to six inches, slender and pale yellow, arising from the axils of the leaves. The catkins arising from the lower leaf axils are entirely male and have eight to ten stamens surrounded by a calyx of five to six green sepals. The ripe pollen has sickly scent. The female flowers are fewer in number and grow in clusters of two or three in a four-lobed involucre (a number of bracts enclosing several flowers) at the base of the catkins in the axils of the upper leaves. The calyx closely surrounds a tapering ovary, at the top of which are five to six radiating stigmas. The involucre later joins together to form the thick leathery hull which covers the ripening seeds – the edible chestnut.

Blooms: later than most trees from June to August, in open woods.

Prepare: by the boiling method. Gather about six inches of the twig with leaves, male and female flowers from as many trees as possible.

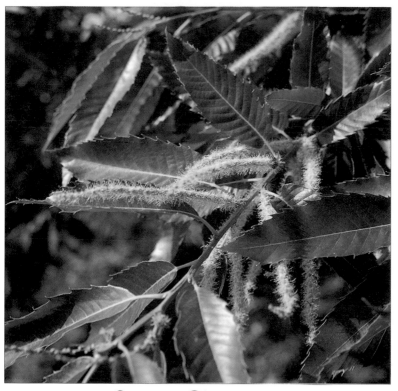

Sweet Chestnut
Castanea sativa

Wild Rose

Indication: for resignation and apathy.

Rosa canina. Dog Rose.

Shrub or bush: four to five feet high, with long arching and prickly branches. The thorns or prickles are equal and hooked.

Leaves: are alternate and broken up into five to seven sharply toothed leaflets, usually in two or three pairs with one terminal leaf, oval in shape. The leaf stalk is joined to the stem by a large two-lobed stipule.

Flowers: white, pink or deep rosy-pink, are either solitary or grow three or four together at the ends of the branches with long stalks. The petals are five in number, notched, large and heart-shaped. The stamens are numerous, and the styles free and hairy . The sepals are five, pinnate, and when the flower opens, they turn downwards towards the stem. The fruit is the "hip" which when ripe, is deep red.

Blooms: from June to August, and grows in thickets, hedges and the fringes of woodlands.

Prepare: by the boiling method. Gather the flowers with a short piece of the stem and leaves from as many bushes as possible. Fill the saucepan three parts full.

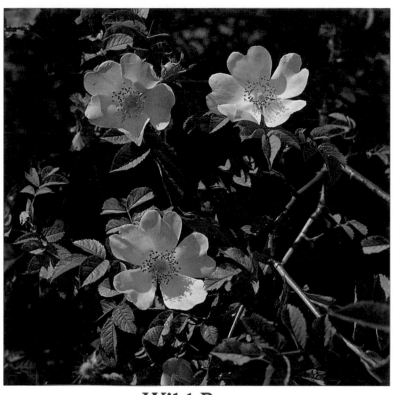

Wild Rose

Rosa canina

Preparing Stock Bottles and Treatment Bottles

The stock bottle is the second stage in the preparation of the remedy and it is from this that the treatment is made up.

To prepare a stock bottle, first fill a sterilized one ounce dropper bottle with brandy. Add two drops from the Tincture bottle of the remedy. Replace cap securely and label with the name of the remedy and "stock".

The treatment bottle is the third stage in the preparation and it is from this that the required daily doses are taken.

After deciding which remedy or combination of remedies are required, put two drops from each into a sterilized one ounce dropper bottle. Fill this with pure spring or mineral water (available in bottles from most supermarkets or health stores), and a teaspoon of brandy to help preserve the water if it is likely to be subjected to a warm environment. Replace the cap securely and label "treatment".

From the treatment bottle, the person takes four drops, four times daily – in a tablespoon of water or fruit juice, first thing in the morning, last thing at night, and twice during the day.

To gain the full effect, the dose should be held in the mouth a moment or so before swallowing.

When necessary, the doses can be given more frequently, every quarter or half hourly, and then hourly until the person feels calmer and more peaceful.

For those who find it difficult to make up a treatment bottle in this way, the treatment can be prepared in a glass of water instead, to be sipped at intervals throughout the day.

NB. Full directions for use available from the Bach Centre.